90 Days of Inspiration

Study Companion for
Social Workers Taking Their Licensing Exams

By Shara Ruffin LCSW

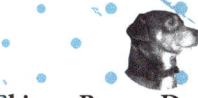

Skinny Brown Dog Media
www.SkinnyBrownDogMedia.com

Published by Skinny Brown Dog Media
Atlanta, Punta del Este
http://www.SkinnyBrownDogMedia.com

Distributed by Skinny Brown Dog Media
Cover Design by Skinny Brown Dog Media

Print ISBN 978-1-957506-08-1

New King James Version is the source file for all Bible quotes, unless otherwise noted

90 Days of Inspiration may be purchased in bulk for educational,business,fundraising
For information,please email SharaRuffin@gmail.com

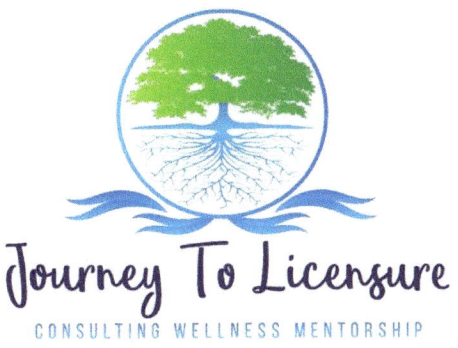

THIS JOURNAL BELONGS TO:

Introduction

Welcome to 90 Days of Inspiration: A Study Companion for Social Workers Taking Their Licensing Exams. This journal was inspired by my decade long journey to get my LCSW (Licensed Clinical Social Worker) license.

I experienced many hardships and life events during those ten years that could have deterred me from getting my license including having a still born daughter; failed military marriage; post-partum depression; generalized anxiety disorder; attention deficit disorder; learning disability; failing my master level licensure exam the first time. I missed the LSW exam by three points. I failed LCSW exam the first time by two points.

When I took my LCSW exam the second time, I kept a journal with positive messages that I wrote to myself during the preparation of my examination process over the course of 90 Days as a coping mechanism to help me cultivate and maintain a positive mindset during the study process.

I hope that with this journal, you are able to stay encouraged in your study process each day.

Sincerely,

Shara Ruffin, LCSW, ACSW, C-SWHC, BC-TMH

> "Believe in yourself and your abilities first and everything else will follow."

DATE: _____ / _____ / _____

Today I am grateful for...

_____

_____

_____

_____

_____

_____

I need to make some adjustments to....

_____

_____

_____

_____

_____

_____

My goal for tomorrow is....

_____

_____

_____

_____

_____

> "Even when you're tired, keep going".
> "Even when you're lonely, Keep going."
> "Even when you feel like you can't go any further, keep going."
> "It is in these moments where you gain the reason. Why you must keep going."
> "Get The Pass".

DATE: _____ / _____ / _____

Today I am grateful for...

_____

_____

_____

_____

_____

I need to make some adjustments to....

_____

_____

_____

_____

_____

_____

My goal for tomorrow is....

_____

_____

_____

_____

_____

> *"Without rain nothing grows, plant those seeds every day, get to work and study."*

DATE: _____ / _____ / _____

Today I am grateful for...

_____

_____

_____

_____

_____

_____

I need to make some adjustments to....

_____

_____

_____

_____

_____

_____

My goal for tomorrow is....

_____

_____

_____

_____

_____

_____

"Believe in yourself first and everything else will follow."

DATE: _____ / _____ / _____

Today I am grateful for...

_____

_____

_____

_____

_____

_____

I need to make some adjustments to....

_____

_____

_____

_____

_____

_____

My goal for tomorrow is....

_____

_____

_____

_____

_____

_____

DATE: _____ / ____ / ____

Today I am grateful for...

_____

_____

_____

_____

_____

I need to make some adjustments to....

_____

_____

_____

_____

_____

My goal for tomorrow is....

_____

_____

_____

_____

_____

"Endure the pain of your study process and enjoy the gain of your outcome, which is your social work license."

DATE: _____ / _____ / _____

Today I am grateful for...

_____
_____
_____
_____
_____
_____

I need to make some adjustments to....

_____
_____
_____
_____
_____
_____
_____

My goal for tomorrow is....

_____
_____
_____
_____
_____
_____

"Each day that you woke is a new apportuity to take a step forward."

DATE: _____ / _____ / _____

Today I am grateful for...

_____

_____

_____

_____

_____

_____

I need to make some adjustments to....

_____

_____

_____

_____

_____

_____

_____

My goal for tomorrow is....

_____

_____

_____

_____

_____

_____

"The best view comes after the hardest climb. Remember that each day of your study process and licensing journey."

DATE: _____ / _____ / _____

Today I am grateful for...

_____

_____

_____

_____

_____

_____

I need to make some adjustments to....

_____

_____

_____

_____

_____

_____

My goal for tomorrow is....

_____

_____

_____

_____

_____

_____

"Change is inevitable, growth is optional. Choose to grow in faith. Choose to grow in your journey. Choose to grow through your fear. Choose to grow during your study process."

DATE: _____ / _____ / _____

Today I am grateful for...

_____
_____
_____
_____
_____
_____

I need to make some adjustments to....

_____
_____
_____
_____
_____
_____
_____

My goal for tomorrow is....

_____
_____
_____
_____
_____
_____

"Each day is another chance to create a new path."

DATE: _____ / ___ / _____

Today I am grateful for...

_____

_____

_____

_____

_____

I need to make some adjustments to....

_____

_____

_____

_____

_____

_____

My goal for tomorrow is....

_____

_____

_____

_____

_____

_____

"Life is a journey, so is your study process, as you move through each phase of your process, remember you will have your good moments and bad moments, take those moments as they come, each moment, each day, has its own lessons. Extract them. Learn from them and move forward."

DATE: _____ / ___ / _____

Today I am grateful for...

_____
_____
_____
_____
_____
_____

I need to make some adjustments to....

_____
_____
_____
_____
_____
_____

My goal for tomorrow is....

_____
_____
_____
_____
_____

"If you want to fly, let go of everything and everyone that weighs you down. Stick with your process."

DATE: _____ / _____ / _____

Today I am grateful for...

_____

_____

_____

_____

_____

_____

I need to make some adjustments to....

_____

_____

_____

_____

_____

_____

My goal for tomorrow is....

_____

_____

_____

_____

_____

_____

"Self-awreness opers doors."

DATE: _____ / _____ / _____

Today I am grateful for...

_____

_____

_____

_____

_____

_____

I need to make some adjustments to....

_____

_____

_____

_____

_____

_____

_____

My goal for tomorrow is....

_____

_____

_____

_____

_____

_____

"Appreciate the dark moments, even you can't see through them yet, they will birth your new beginning if you listen to the lessors that they will cultivate for you, use those lessons as your blueprint to ace your exam and get licensed."

DATE: _____ / _____ / _____

Today I am grateful for...

_____

_____

_____

_____

_____

_____

I need to make some adjustments to....

_____

_____

_____

_____

_____

_____

My goal for tomorrow is....

_____

_____

_____

_____

_____

_____

> "*Believe in yourself. Believe in your capacity to do great things. Believe that no storm is so great that you cannot weather it you can weather the study process of your exams.*"

DATE: _____ / ____ / _____

Today I am grateful for...

_____

_____

_____

_____

_____

_____

I need to make some adjustments to....

_____

_____

_____

_____

_____

_____

My goal for tomorrow is....

_____

_____

_____

_____

_____

> *"Confidence is half the battle, keep moving forward despite your internal battle with yourself."*

DATE: _____ / _____ / _____

Today I am grateful for...

_____
_____
_____
_____
_____

I need to make some adjustments to....

_____
_____
_____
_____
_____

My goal for tomorrow is....

_____
_____
_____
_____
_____

"You learn more from failure than from success. Don't let it stop you. Failure builds character. No matter many times you have taken this exam, know that there is a lesson, a blessing in the failure, learn from it and keep moving forward. Remember, someone is waiting for you to pass. To bless them with your social work gifts. Get the pass."

DATE: _____ / _____ / _____

Today I am grateful for...

_____

_____

_____

_____

_____

I need to make some adjustments to....

_____

_____

_____

_____

_____

_____

My goal for tomorrow is....

_____

_____

_____

_____

_____

"This is your season. It is your time. The past is your lesson, The present is your gift, The future is your motivation. The social work license is your future, now make it a reality."

DATE: _____ / ____ / _____

Today I am grateful for...

_____
_____
_____
_____
_____
_____

I need to make some adjustments to....

_____
_____
_____
_____
_____
_____

My goal for tomorrow is....

_____
_____
_____
_____
_____
_____

"If you don't try, you won't start.
Just start and the rest will come."

DATE: _____ / ____ / ____

Today I am grateful for...

_____

_____

_____

_____

_____

_____

I need to make some adjustments to....

_____

_____

_____

_____

_____

_____

My goal for tomorrow is....

_____

_____

_____

_____

_____

_____

> *"You can do amazing things when you believe in yourself and your process."*

DATE: _____ / _____ / _____

Today I am grateful for...

_____

_____

_____

_____

_____

I need to make some adjustments to....

_____

_____

_____

_____

_____

My goal for tomorrow is....

_____

_____

_____

_____

_____

DATE: _____ / ___ / ___

Today I am grateful for...

_____

_____

_____

_____

_____

_____

I need to make some adjustments to....

_____

_____

_____

_____

_____

_____

My goal for tomorrow is....

_____

_____

_____

_____

_____

_____

"Don't compare your journey to someone else's journey. Everyone's journey is different."

DATE: _____ / _____ / _____

Today I am grateful for...

_____

_____

_____

_____

_____

_____

I need to make some adjustments to....

_____

_____

_____

_____

_____

_____

My goal for tomorrow is....

_____

_____

_____

_____

_____

_____

"Every day is a new opportunity to get that license, grind those study hours out and get that pass, no matter what happened yesterday."

DATE: _____ / ___ / _____

Today I am grateful for...

_____

_____

_____

_____

_____

_____

I need to make some adjustments to....

_____

_____

_____

_____

_____

_____

My goal for tomorrow is....

_____

_____

_____

_____

_____

_____

> *"The more consistent you are with taking care of yourself, the more consistent your outcomes will be. Self care is pivotal during your study process."*

DATE: _____ / _____ / _____

Today I am grateful for...

_____

_____

_____

_____

_____

_____

I need to make some adjustments to....

_____

_____

_____

_____

_____

_____

My goal for tomorrow is....

_____

_____

_____

_____

_____

> *"Win the battle in your mind first, it's the toughest battle there is."*

DATE: _____ / ___ / ___

Today I am grateful for...

_____

_____

_____

_____

_____

I need to make some adjustments to....

_____

_____

_____

_____

_____

_____

My goal for tomorrow is....

_____

_____

_____

_____

_____

"Life goes on whether you choose to move with it and take a chance on an unknown path or stay behind locked into your past, thinking of what could have been. You have the power to choose. Choose wisely. Get that pass."

DATE: _____ / ____ / _____

Today I am grateful for...

_____

_____

_____

_____

_____

_____

I need to make some adjustments to....

_____

_____

_____

_____

_____

_____

My goal for tomorrow is....

_____

_____

_____

_____

_____

"Trust the wait. Embrace the uncertainty. Enjoy the beauty of becoming. When nothing is certain, anything is possible."

DATE: _____ / _____ / _____

Today I am grateful for...

_____
_____
_____
_____
_____
_____

I need to make some adjustments to....

_____
_____
_____
_____
_____
_____

My goal for tomorrow is....

_____
_____
_____
_____
_____
_____

"You are the only one that can cultivate the win.
Get The Pass!"

DATE: _____ / _____ / _____

Today I am grateful for...

_____

_____

_____

_____

_____

_____

I need to make some adjustments to....

_____

_____

_____

_____

_____

_____

My goal for tomorrow is....

_____

_____

_____

_____

_____

_____

_____

*"Push yourself because no one else is going to do it for you.
Get The Pass!"*

DATE: _____ / ____ / ____

Today I am grateful for...

_____

_____

_____

_____

_____

I need to make some adjustments to....

_____

_____

_____

_____

_____

My goal for tomorrow is....

_____

_____

_____

_____

_____

> *"Let go of what is gone, be grateful for what remains, look forward to what is to come. Get the pass."*

DATE: _____ / ___ / _____

Today I am grateful for...

_____

_____

_____

_____

_____

_____

I need to make some adjustments to....

_____

_____

_____

_____

_____

_____

My goal for tomorrow is....

_____

_____

_____

_____

_____

_____

"Open that study guide and get to work, one day your hard work will pay off and will result in a pass on that test screen. The sooner you get started the faster you will have a result."

DATE: _____ / _____ / _____

Today I am grateful for...

_____

_____

_____

_____

_____

_____

I need to make some adjustments to....

_____

_____

_____

_____

_____

_____

My goal for tomorrow is....

_____

_____

_____

_____

_____

"Life is short. Live it. Fear is natural, Make it temporary. Face it. Memory is powerful. Use it. Now get the studying."

DATE: _____ / ___ / _____

Today I am grateful for...

_____

_____

_____

_____

_____

_____

I need to make some adjustments to....

_____

_____

_____

_____

_____

My goal for tomorrow is....

_____

_____

_____

_____

_____

"Do what is right, not what is easy.
Get to work."

DATE: _____ / ____ / ____

Today I am grateful for...

_____

_____

_____

_____

_____

_____

I need to make some adjustments to....

_____

_____

_____

_____

_____

_____

My goal for tomorrow is....

_____

_____

_____

_____

_____

_____

> *"We generate fears while we do nothing. We overcome these fears by taking action. Start the study process today."*

DATE: _____ / ___ / _____

Today I am grateful for...

_____

_____

_____

_____

_____

_____

I need to make some adjustments to....

_____

_____

_____

_____

_____

_____

My goal for tomorrow is....

_____

_____

_____

_____

_____

_____

> "It's never too late to be what you might have been.
> Get the pass."

DATE: _____ / ___ / ___

Today I am grateful for...

_____
_____
_____
_____
_____
_____

I need to make some adjustments to....

_____
_____
_____
_____
_____
_____

My goal for tomorrow is....

_____
_____
_____
_____
_____
_____

DATE: _____ / ____ / _____

Today I am grateful for...

_____
_____
_____
_____
_____
_____

I need to make some adjustments to....

_____
_____
_____
_____
_____
_____

My goal for tomorrow is....

_____
_____
_____
_____
_____
_____

"You don't have to be great to start. But you have to start to be great. Get the pass."

DATE: _____ / _____ / _____

Today I am grateful for...

_____

_____

_____

_____

_____

_____

I need to make some adjustments to....

_____

_____

_____

_____

_____

_____

My goal for tomorrow is....

_____

_____

_____

_____

_____

_____

"Every morning you have two choices: continue to sleep with your dreams, or wake up and chase them."

DATE: _____ / _____ / _____

Today I am grateful for...

_____
_____
_____
_____
_____

I need to make some adjustments to....

_____
_____
_____
_____
_____
_____

My goal for tomorrow is....

_____
_____
_____
_____
_____
_____

"You have to visualize your self passing the test, Plant the seed in your mind and it will grow in reality."

DATE: _____ / _____ / _____

Today I am grateful for...

_____

_____

_____

_____

_____

_____

I need to make some adjustments to....

_____

_____

_____

_____

_____

_____

My goal for tomorrow is....

_____

_____

_____

_____

_____

_____

> *"The road to success is your resilence*
> *to stay the course."*

DATE: _____ / _____ / _____

Today I am grateful for...

_____
_____
_____
_____
_____
_____

I need to make some adjustments to....

_____
_____
_____
_____
_____
_____

My goal for tomorrow is....

_____
_____
_____
_____
_____
_____

"Don't let the ghost of your past keep you from the blessings of your future."

DATE: _____ / _____ / _____

Today I am grateful for...

_____

_____

_____

_____

_____

I need to make some adjustments to....

_____

_____

_____

_____

_____

My goal for tomorrow is....

_____

_____

_____

_____

_____

"As long as we press forward through the storms of life, we will have our chance in the sun. Keep studying !!!! You can do this!"

DATE: _____ / _____ / _____

Today I am grateful for...

_____
_____
_____
_____
_____
_____

I need to make some adjustments to....

_____
_____
_____
_____
_____
_____

My goal for tomorrow is....

_____
_____
_____
_____
_____
_____

"I have done everything I could during my study process to pass my exam. I will trust in my abilities."

DATE: _____ / ____ / ____

Today I am grateful for...

_____
_____
_____
_____
_____
_____

I need to make some adjustments to....

_____
_____
_____
_____
_____
_____

My goal for tomorrow is....

_____
_____
_____
_____
_____
_____

> *"A little progress each day, adds up to big results!*
> *Keep going! Period!"*

DATE: _____ / _____ / _____

Today I am grateful for...

_____

_____

_____

_____

_____

_____

I need to make some adjustments to....

_____

_____

_____

_____

_____

_____

My goal for tomorrow is....

_____

_____

_____

_____

_____

_____

"Focus on where you want to go, not where you are currently. Where you focus on your future, it becomes reality."

DATE: _____ / _____ / _____

Today I am grateful for...

_____

_____

_____

_____

_____

I need to make some adjustments to....

_____

_____

_____

_____

_____

_____

My goal for tomorrow is....

_____

_____

_____

_____

_____

"Failure is not fatal."

DATE: _____ / _____ / _____

Today I am grateful for...

_____

_____

_____

_____

_____

_____

I need to make some adjustments to....

_____

_____

_____

_____

_____

_____

My goal for tomorrow is....

_____

_____

_____

_____

_____

_____

"You are the biggest investment you will ever make, be consistent and intentional in your study process."

DATE: _____ / _____ / _____

Today I am grateful for...

_____

_____

_____

_____

_____

_____

I need to make some adjustments to....

_____

_____

_____

_____

_____

_____

My goal for tomorrow is....

_____

_____

_____

_____

_____

_____

DATE: _____ / _____ / _____

Today I am grateful for...

_____
_____
_____
_____
_____
_____

I need to make some adjustments to....

_____
_____
_____
_____
_____
_____

My goal for tomorrow is....

_____
_____
_____
_____
_____
_____

"You didn't come this far just to stop, often when we just feel like giving up, we are closer to accomplishing our goal than we think. Keep going!"

DATE: _____ / ____ / ____

Today I am grateful for...

_____

_____

_____

_____

_____

_____

I need to make some adjustments to....

_____

_____

_____

_____

_____

_____

My goal for tomorrow is....

_____

_____

_____

_____

_____

_____

> "Each day the sunrises is another day to work on your goals. Never give up !"

DATE: ___ / ___ / ___

Today I am grateful for...

_____
_____
_____
_____
_____
_____

I need to make some adjustments to....

_____
_____
_____
_____
_____
_____

My goal for tomorrow is....

_____
_____
_____
_____
_____
_____

DATE: _____ / _____ / _____

Today I am grateful for...

_____

_____

_____

_____

_____

_____

I need to make some adjustments to....

_____

_____

_____

_____

_____

_____

My goal for tomorrow is....

_____

_____

_____

_____

_____

> "When you feel like giving up, remember why you held on in the first place."

DATE: _____ / _____ / _____

Today I am grateful for...

_____

_____

_____

_____

_____

_____

I need to make some adjustments to....

_____

_____

_____

_____

_____

_____

My goal for tomorrow is....

_____

_____

_____

_____

_____

_____

DATE: _____ / ____ / ____

Today I am grateful for...

_____

_____

_____

_____

_____

_____

I need to make some adjustments to....

_____

_____

_____

_____

_____

_____

My goal for tomorrow is....

_____

_____

_____

_____

_____

_____

"Your only limit is you."

DATE: _____ / _____ / _____

Today I am grateful for...

_____

_____

_____

_____

_____

_____

I need to make some adjustments to....

_____

_____

_____

_____

_____

_____

My goal for tomorrow is....

_____

_____

_____

_____

_____

_____

DATE: _____ / ___ / ___

Today I am grateful for...

_____

_____

_____

_____

_____

_____

I need to make some adjustments to....

_____

_____

_____

_____

_____

_____

My goal for tomorrow is....

_____

_____

_____

_____

_____

"I'm too tired after work to study. Many things are not equal but everyone gets the same 24 hours a day, 7 days a week. We make time for what we truly want. Switch up your plan if you have to. Don't give up."

DATE: _____ / _____ / _____

Today I am grateful for...

_____

_____

_____

_____

_____

_____

I need to make some adjustments to....

_____

_____

_____

_____

_____

_____

My goal for tomorrow is....

_____

_____

_____

_____

_____

_____

"In order to get what you never had, you have to do something you never did, to get a different result."

DATE: _____ / ____ / ____

Today I am grateful for...

_____

_____

_____

_____

_____

_____

I need to make some adjustments to....

_____

_____

_____

_____

_____

_____

My goal for tomorrow is....

_____

_____

_____

_____

_____

_____

"Feeling unmotivated? Think of why you want this license. What is your vision for yourself and where it gets hard, hold on to the vision, now go put the work in."

DATE: _____ / ___ / _____

Today I am grateful for...

_____
_____
_____
_____
_____
_____

I need to make some adjustments to....

_____
_____
_____
_____
_____
_____

My goal for tomorrow is....

_____
_____
_____
_____
_____
_____

> *"Look at every setback as a sign from the universe on how to move forward in a new and more aligned way, don't quit, keep going forward."*

DATE: _____ / _____ / _____

Today I am grateful for...

_____
_____
_____
_____
_____
_____

I need to make some adjustments to....

_____
_____
_____
_____
_____
_____

My goal for tomorrow is....

_____
_____
_____
_____
_____

"Remember take it one day at a time."

DATE: _____ / _____ / _____

Today I am grateful for...

_____

_____

_____

_____

_____

_____

I need to make some adjustments to....

_____

_____

_____

_____

_____

_____

My goal for tomorrow is....

_____

_____

_____

_____

_____

_____

"

"Stay true to your own process and trust that it will lead you in the direction you need to go."

DATE: _____ / _____ / _____

Today I am grateful for...

_____

_____

_____

_____

_____

_____

I need to make some adjustments to....

_____

_____

_____

_____

_____

_____

My goal for tomorrow is....

_____

_____

_____

_____

_____

"For every door that closes, for every attempt to climb, hardship, struggle has a purpose."

DATE: _____ / _____ / _____

Today I am grateful for...

_____

_____

_____

_____

_____

_____

I need to make some adjustments to....

_____

_____

_____

_____

_____

_____

My goal for tomorrow is....

_____

_____

_____

_____

_____

_____

> "*Don't second guess yourself when it comes to practice questions, listen to your intuition and keep it moving.*"

DATE: _____ / _____ / _____

Today I am grateful for...

_____

_____

_____

_____

_____

_____

I need to make some adjustments to....

_____

_____

_____

_____

_____

_____

_____

My goal for tomorrow is....

_____

_____

_____

_____

_____

_____

> "There are seven days in a week and someday isn't one of them, Get to studying!."

DATE: _____ / _____ / _____

Today I am grateful for...

_____
_____
_____
_____
_____
_____

I need to make some adjustments to....

_____
_____
_____
_____
_____
_____

My goal for tomorrow is....

_____
_____
_____
_____
_____
_____

"Life begins at the end of your comfort zone. Do something different in your study process if needed. But don't stop your process."

DATE: _____ / ___ / ___

Today I am grateful for...

_____
_____
_____
_____
_____

I need to make some adjustments to....

_____
_____
_____
_____
_____

My goal for tomorrow is....

_____
_____
_____
_____
_____

"Do not look at how long it will take you to accomplish those goals or how hard it will be, take it, step by step and know that one day it will all be worth it."

DATE: _____ / _____ / _____

Today I am grateful for...

_____

_____

_____

_____

_____

_____

I need to make some adjustments to....

_____

_____

_____

_____

_____

_____

_____

My goal for tomorrow is....

_____

_____

_____

_____

_____

_____

"Success requires daily action."

DATE: _____ / _____ / _____

Today I am grateful for...

_____

_____

_____

_____

_____

_____

I need to make some adjustments to....

_____

_____

_____

_____

_____

_____

My goal for tomorrow is....

_____

_____

_____

_____

_____

DATE: _____ / ___ / _____

Today I am grateful for...

_____

_____

_____

_____

_____

I need to make some adjustments to....

_____

_____

_____

_____

_____

_____

My goal for tomorrow is....

_____

_____

_____

_____

_____

_____

"Live less out of habit and more out of intent."

DATE: _____ / ____ / ____

Today I am grateful for...

_____

_____

_____

_____

_____

_____

I need to make some adjustments to....

_____

_____

_____

_____

_____

_____

My goal for tomorrow is....

_____

_____

_____

_____

_____

_____

> *"When you focus on faith rather than fear, you tap into a strength to carry you over the tallest mountain."*

DATE: _____ / _____ / _____

Today I am grateful for...

_____

_____

_____

_____

_____

_____

I need to make some adjustments to....

_____

_____

_____

_____

_____

_____

My goal for tomorrow is....

_____

_____

_____

_____

_____

_____

> # "
> *"Be a dreamer, who dares to make it real.*
> *Get that license!"*

DATE: _____ / _____ / _____

Today I am grateful for...

_____
_____
_____
_____
_____
_____

I need to make some adjustments to....

_____
_____
_____
_____
_____
_____

My goal for tomorrow is....

_____
_____
_____
_____
_____
_____

"I can and will pass."

DATE: _____ / _____ / _____

Today I am grateful for...

_____

_____

_____

_____

_____

_____

I need to make some adjustments to....

_____

_____

_____

_____

_____

_____

My goal for tomorrow is....

_____

_____

_____

_____

_____

"The best way out is through. Get the studying process in."

DATE: _____ / ____ / ____

Today I am grateful for...

_____

_____

_____

_____

_____

I need to make some adjustments to....

_____

_____

_____

_____

_____

_____

My goal for tomorrow is....

_____

_____

_____

_____

_____

> *"Keep going. Everything you need will come at the perfect time."*

DATE: _____ / ____ / ____

Today I am grateful for...

_____

_____

_____

_____

_____

I need to make some adjustments to....

_____

_____

_____

_____

_____

My goal for tomorrow is....

_____

_____

_____

_____

_____

> *"Start where you are. Use what you have. Do what you can."*

DATE: _____ / _____ / _____

Today I am grateful for...

_____
_____
_____
_____
_____

I need to make some adjustments to....

_____
_____
_____
_____
_____

My goal for tomorrow is....

_____
_____
_____
_____
_____

> ## "Dont be afraid to fail,
> ## be afraid not to try."

DATE: _____ / _____ / _____

Today I am grateful for...

_____

_____

_____

_____

_____

_____

I need to make some adjustments to....

_____

_____

_____

_____

_____

_____

My goal for tomorrow is....

_____

_____

_____

_____

_____

_____

> *"The day you plant the seed is not the day you eat the fruit.*
> *Keep studying, Keep going period."*

DATE: _____ / ___ / ___

Today I am grateful for...

_____
_____
_____
_____
_____

I need to make some adjustments to....

_____
_____
_____
_____
_____

My goal for tomorrow is....

_____
_____
_____
_____
_____

"Invest in rest, along your journey, it doesn't mean stop studying, but take breaks where needed in your process."

DATE: _____ / _____ / _____

Today I am grateful for...

_____

_____

_____

_____

_____

_____

I need to make some adjustments to....

_____

_____

_____

_____

_____

_____

My goal for tomorrow is....

_____

_____

_____

_____

_____

_____

> *"Strength grows in the moments, when you think you can't go on but you keep going anyway."*

DATE: _____ / _____ / _____

Today I am grateful for...

_____

_____

_____

_____

_____

_____

I need to make some adjustments to....

_____

_____

_____

_____

_____

_____

My goal for tomorrow is....

_____

_____

_____

_____

_____

"Small steps of discipline repeated with consistency every day, lead to great achievements gained slowly over time."

DATE: _____ / _____ / _____

Today I am grateful for...

_____
_____
_____
_____
_____
_____

I need to make some adjustments to....

_____
_____
_____
_____
_____
_____

My goal for tomorrow is....

_____
_____
_____
_____
_____

"Feed the positive, starve the negative."

DATE: _____ / _____ / _____

Today I am grateful for...

_____

_____

_____

_____

_____

_____

I need to make some adjustments to....

_____

_____

_____

_____

_____

_____

My goal for tomorrow is....

_____

_____

_____

_____

_____

DATE: _____ / ____ / ____

Today I am grateful for...

_____
_____
_____
_____
_____
_____

I need to make some adjustments to....

_____
_____
_____
_____
_____
_____

My goal for tomorrow is....

_____
_____
_____
_____
_____
_____

DATE: _____ / _____ / _____

Today I am grateful for...

_____

_____

_____

_____

_____

_____

I need to make some adjustments to....

_____

_____

_____

_____

_____

_____

_____

My goal for tomorrow is....

_____

_____

_____

_____

_____

_____

> "To change your life, you have to change your priorities. Protect and prioritize your study time."

DATE: _____ / _____ / _____

Today I am grateful for...

_____

_____

_____

_____

_____

_____

I need to make some adjustments to....

_____

_____

_____

_____

_____

_____

My goal for tomorrow is....

_____

_____

_____

_____

_____

_____

DATE: _____ / _____ / _____

Today I am grateful for...

_____

_____

_____

_____

_____

_____

I need to make some adjustments to....

_____

_____

_____

_____

_____

_____

My goal for tomorrow is....

_____

_____

_____

_____

_____

_____

"Be mindful of your self-talk, for it is the conversation that becomes your reality. Keep feeding yourself positive thoughts in your study process."

DATE: _____ / _____ / _____

Today I am grateful for...

_____
_____
_____
_____
_____

I need to make some adjustments to....

_____
_____
_____
_____
_____

My goal for tomorrow is....

_____
_____
_____
_____
_____

> *"Never allow waiting to become a habit. The perfect time will rarely come. Life is happening now, take a step forward. Get your license. Go study!"*

DATE: _____ / _____ / _____

Today I am grateful for...

_____

_____

_____

_____

_____

_____

I need to make some adjustments to....

_____

_____

_____

_____

_____

_____

My goal for tomorrow is....

_____

_____

_____

_____

_____

"You are taking steps, even when you feel like it's just one step. Remember one step forward is better than no steps at all. Take control over your journey and study are day at a time."

DATE: _____ / _____ / _____

Today I am grateful for...

_____
_____
_____
_____
_____
_____

I need to make some adjustments to....

_____
_____
_____
_____
_____

My goal for tomorrow is....

_____
_____
_____
_____
_____
_____

"Faith it until you make it."

DATE: _____ / ___ / ___

Today I am grateful for...

_____

_____

_____

_____

_____

_____

I need to make some adjustments to....

_____

_____

_____

_____

_____

_____

My goal for tomorrow is....

_____

_____

_____

_____

_____

"Take it one day at a time, one hour at a time, one minute at a time, one second at a time. Remember Rome was not built in a day."

DATE: _____ / _____ / _____

Today I am grateful for...

_____

_____

_____

_____

_____

_____

I need to make some adjustments to....

_____

_____

_____

_____

_____

_____

My goal for tomorrow is....

_____

_____

_____

_____

_____

Journal

Journal

Journal

Journal

Journal

Journal

Lightning Source UK Ltd.
Milton Keynes UK
UKHW050636090822
407046UK00005B/66

9 781957 506081